Still Dancing Through Life

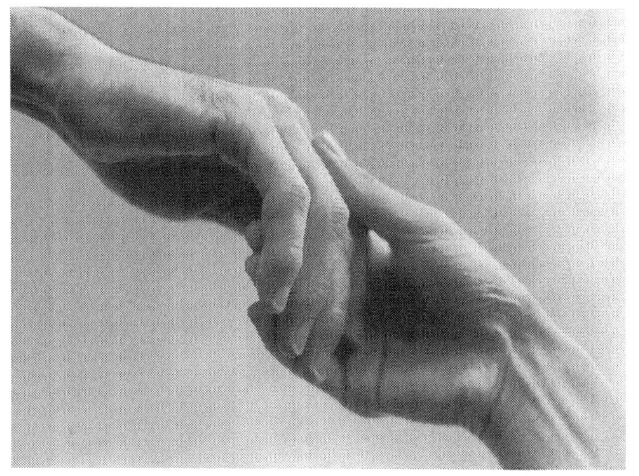

A Love Story

Dr. Gretchen Helm

iUniverse, Inc.
Bloomington

Still Dancing Through Life
A Love Story

iUniverse books may be ordered through booksellers or by contacting:

iUniverse
1663 Liberty Drive
Bloomington, IN 47403
www.iuniverse.com
1-800-Authors (1-800-288-4677)

ISBN: 978-1-4759-3738-1 (sc)
ISBN: 978-1-4759-3739-8 (ebk)

Printed in the United States of America

iUniverse rev. date: 07/12/2012

Contents

For Norm

Again

Acknowledgements

There are countless numbers of caregivers whose devotion to the people they care for is a testament to the power of love. These people give new meaning to the words: commitment and sacrifice.

My husband, Norm Helm, is in assisted living, and as I visit him, I have found that our love for each other deepens and grows richer with each passing day. I also have the great privilege of seeing family members remain steadfast in the care of their loved ones. They let them know each time they see them that they're not forgotten and never will be.

Unfortunately, most caregivers, many without help and support, don't have the means to have the person they are caring for be part of an assisted living community, but through love they persevere. I hope they know how very special they are.

In assisted living there are staff members who caretake residents with Alzheimer's or dementia, of which there are many types. These caretakers deal with the most difficult situations one could imagine and do so day after day. As a result, the residents are always clean, well fed, treated with respect and are safe from harm. There are those, too, who make the facility run smoothly and care for the needs of both the residents and their families.

Dr. Gretchen Helm

To Lesley, Ann, B.J., Pamela, Lisa, Iva, Betty, Judi, Doris, Stephanie, Nate, Helen, Robert, Craig, Loretta and all the other caretakers in this and every other assisted living facility, I greatly admire your patience, your compassion, and your loving care for the residents you serve. You have enriched both my husband's and my life.

Not all angels have wings.

Introduction

"May you have an interesting life" is a Chinese curse. Somehow, somewhere I was the recipient of that curse. I don't even know any Chinese people. It could have been that Chinese waiter at Ning Wa, although I'm pretty sure I gave him a decent tip. Maybe it was from another life. I'm beginning to believe what Shirley McLaine says about reincarnation. I might have been a Chinese coolie who somehow offended someone I worked with in the rice fields, and now I'm doomed to live an interesting life. I wonder if this curse transfers into my future reincarnations. I'm going to seek me out a Chinese person and get the scoop on this curse. It sure doesn't seem fair, but then again I never thought it was fair to spend $.25 on the Chinese finger thing that got tighter and tighter as you tried to remove your fingers. How was I to know that all you had to do was to relax and put your fingers closer together and wa la (that's Chinese for "Who knew?") blessed release. Maybe that's how I should deal with this curse; just relax and be released. Nah! That's too simple. I'd rather fight it. It takes my mind off my problems.

My first marriage was a challenge as my husband had health issues that put an enormous strain on our marriage. As in most marriages, there are problems; some that can be resolved and others that cannot. We had two children, Lori and Kris. When things got difficult, and I didn't think I could keep on going, I loaded all my things and the girls into my Volkswagen and just sat in the driveway. I had nowhere to go, so we went nowhere but back into the house. This was true of many women of my generation that had to endure unhappy marriages, not having the resources to do otherwise. After seventeen years, no matter what the consequences as I didn't have a job or any financial resources, I filed for divorce and became a single mother doing my best to survive and to make the best lives possible for my girls.

Then came a guy who proved to be anything but "interesting" (interesting as in the Chinese curse). He was the pastor of a the Congregational church in Westborough, MA. He was admired and respected by all who knew him. We got married. Now I could look forward to a normal, stable family life for probably the first time in my life. Unlike my family of origin, there would be no more turkeys thrown against the wall on Thanksgiving and being brought to dinner at the Fish and Game Club under the threat of my father suddenly going bonkers and shooting up the whole place with the pistol he had in his pocket. There are carrots and there are sticks. This definitely was not a carrot.

Now the curse was over. How wonderful to be the wife of the pastor, able to be a cross between Mother Teresa and Bozo the Clown. You have a lot of leeway when you're the wife of the boss. Now my children had the father to fill in the gap as their own father had started a new life and was rarely around. What an ideal situation. How much better could it get. Of course, his children cursed the ground I walked on, but since they were living far enough away, it was never a problem until they flew in on their brooms to put a damper on any holiday when they chose to grant us the pleasure of their company.

So when did the Chinese Curse kick in? It was probably three years after our marriage when blocked arteries led to triple bypass. No big deal. After a brief time of recuperation, Norm was back to work full force. Five years of curse-free living. What a break. Then the curse came back with a vengeance. I guess there's a curse rule that says that if you have a certain amount of time curse-free, you get it back in spades.

Some teenager, not a very experienced driver, left school early and was happily on her way to meet a friend. Unfortunately, her trip was cut short by the simple matter of running the local preacher down in the street. December 1, 1989; a day that will live in infamy. Now the real fun started; life-flight helicopter, hospitalization, three months of rehab, and a future of dealing with traumatic head injury. Needless to say, retirement came early for both of us. The good news was that the year before we had visited New Mexico, fell in love with it and bought a lovely piece of land just below the Sandia Mountains. This was our perfect means to escape and to recover. Again, the curse was put on hold. We had fifteen wonderful, challenging, exciting, years in The Land of Enchantment. Then, in a fit of fear and pique, I decided that it was time to move on to a new life. We had just been robbed, broken into while we were sleeping, and our neighbor built this atrocious addition outside our bedroom window which blocked our view of the lights of the city which I referred to as "Christmas every night without having to pay the electricity bill."

So where did we go? Sight unseen we moved to North Carolina. Not a very smart decision. It was supposed to be a great plan because we would be back on the East Coast close to family and friends. Because of the distance between us, in two years, we had about three visits from the aforementioned family, all of whom were extremely busy, while we languished in bubbaville; a major interesting experience. From the moment we arrived, we realized what a mistake it was to leave New Mexico; our busy lives, our fun and supportive friends, our newfound church, The United Church of Christ, that was accepting of all people.

To take our minds off our unhappiness and self-flagellation about making such an ill-advised move, we were now about to learn the real meaning of "May you have an interesting life." Norm started exhibiting strange, inexplicable behaviors which bordered on being dangerous for us both. Diagnosis: dementia. Norm had now graduated from traumatic brain injury to dementia. Any connection? According to medical research, traumatic brain injury, followed by dementia is a very common thing. How much more interesting can life get? I don't think I want to know as long as there are sharp objects around.

I wasn't one to say, "Why me?" I never said it when I was the recipient of good luck. I sure as heck wasn't going to say it then. However, I did decide to ask God what in the world was going on? It must have been a slow day for him because he decided to answer me. He said, "Okay, I'm going to try to help you understand this. I decided that I was going to go through the alphabet with you. First there was atherosclerosis, which means blocked arteries, which led to triple-bypass surgery.

Then it seemed reasonable to move on to the next challenge: brain injury. After nineteen years of dealing with that, it was time for challenge number 3: dementia."

"Wait a minute I said. Whatever happened to "C"?' Oh, God said '"C" would have to be cancer and that usually has a lot of throwing up that goes with it, and even I can't stand that. So I skipped "C" and went right to "D".' Was I supposed to be grateful? What followed were lots of interesting experiences but no throwing up. How fortunate, and here I was all prepared with a stash of paper towels and a barf bucket. Instead I got the opportunity to meet our local sheriff's department when they brought my husband home from a night of wandering the neighborhood in his underwear.

I had to get out of that place, but the real estate market was so depressed that we couldn't sell our house, which was at a bargain basement price. People were scared. It might have been a buyer's market, but there weren't any buyers. I guess you would call this "the real estate curse." So there we were: stuck. There is nothing worse in the world than being without hope. I guess it's human nature, at least it's my human nature, to plan for the future. A friend once told me, "We plan. God laughs." So how do you live without planning for the future and looking forward to all the wonderful things that await you somewhere down the road? God must be having a real good laugh at all of us planners. Actually, when I thought about it, my last plan was a real doozey; move to North Carolina and start a new life. I waited for the "new life", but it just didn't happen. In the meantime, I was taking the advice of all the wise people who said to live in the moment. I suppose that would work well if your moments were filled with laughter and joy and hope. But what if you just felt stuck? Each of those delicious moments that we were supposed to be enjoying to the fullest seemed to allude us.

And then there's always the uninvited "guest" dementia who decided to move in and take over our lives. Everywhere we turned, he was there. He was the master of confusion and the creator of everything from discomfort to downright misery. We couldn't ask him to leave because we were informed that he was here to stay, like it or not. We couldn't escape him, as hard as we tried. He followed us from room to room. When we got furious at him and his horrible behavior, he just laughed and told us that he was only doing his job. "What's the problem? I'm just making your life more interesting." What a guy. So then all we could do was wait for what he planned to do next to create upheaval in our lives. Our friends and family asked what they could do to help. How about shooting the little devil. Believe me, no one would miss him. Other than that, we just depended upon notes of encouragement, comforting phone calls and lots and lots of prayers. I can just hear God saying, "Give me some credit. I didn't give them the big C. Give me a big break."

How many times have I stood in awe of those people who faced adversity with grace and courage? I always prayed that I could rise to the occasion when the occasion arose, but by then I was wondering *how* to rise. Where was the optimistic person I used to be? It's always darkest before the storm. This too shall pass. Everything happens for a reason. Nothing lasts forever. When I had days of beautiful, merciful denial, I repeated all of those things and more. Then when I fell into a pit of despair and there seemed to be no hope, I became paralyzed with feelings of powerlessness.

There's absolutely nothing I could do to change the situation. There were no magic bullets or magic wands. Dementia was here to stay. Gas prices were out of sight. The real estate market was dead, dead, dead. Then I tried to think of all those people, and there were many, who had it worse than I did. Some people were relieved of their burden of debt by having their homes foreclosed and their cars repossessed. Some people were on chemo and some people couldn't afford chemo because of our horrific healthcare system. Some people lost their children and spent weekends putting flowers on their final resting places. So I guess our new "friend" dementia can be tolerated once in awhile but in small doses. The thing that is so maddening about Mr. dementia is that some days he would be very well behaved. In fact, you wouldn't even know that he was around. Then he would decide to make mischief and create fantasies and delusions. That must have been really fun for him, having the wherewithal to invade someone's mind and churn things up while he sits back and congratulates himself on doing such a great job. I gave up asking him to leave because he'd taken up permanent residence, like it or not.

So life continues to be interesting, and I'm still looking for that damn Chinese person who is sitting back watching his curse unfold. May he have an interesting life.

The Beginning of an Interesting Life

I was born at the beginning of WWII. My father was a member of the National Guard at the time, and when his unit was activated, my father was rejected because he was blind in one eye. He was determined to be part of the effort to win the war, so he went to the Merchant Marines Office and asked how he could join. He was told that there was a hospital ship, The Dogwood, which needed a medical doctor and a cook. My father was always one to bluff his way into or out of something, so he told them that he was a trained cook. He had never cooked a meal in his life, but neither had he treated sick and injured people, so fortunately for all the shipmates, he didn't say that he was a doctor. Phew!

So it was me and my mother; my mother who didn't have a mothering bone in her body. Since my mother had been raised by an aunt who took her in when she was three-years old after her mother died, my aunt took over where my mother left off, which was when I was born. My mother was always self-focused and remained so for all her life—and mine. As a consequence, I was always looking for attention. I got much more than I needed in grade school. I was constantly getting in trouble and ending up in the principal's office. The principal, Miss Eaton, had served in the army, and she was ruthless. She took no prisoners. Every time I was sent to the office, Miss Eaton became more and more annoyed and frustrated with me. I was her least favorite student, to say the least.

One of the perks of being in James B. Crowley grade school was that each week a sixth grade student was chosen to ring the bell when school was to start. They would ring the bell for recess and when recess was over. They would ring the bell at the end of the school day. There were two sixth grade classes, and each week Miss Eaton would enter a classroom and ask who would like to ring the bells the next week. I would always raise my hand along with all the others who hadn't had a chance. By the end of the year, every student in one class had the chance to ring the bells. So now, our class was down to one student who hadn't been given that honor, and that would be me. When Miss Eaton came into the classroom to ask who would like to ring the bells the following week, my hand was the only one to go up. Without hesitation, Miss Eaton said, "Would anyone like to ring the bells a second time?" I was devastated. I would never have a chance to ring the bells. Maybe this fact would follow me throughout my life, and I would be known as the girl who had never been chosen to ring the bells. It was humiliating, and I'm sure it has had a long-lasting affect on my psyche.

To say that my family was dysfunctional would be a gross understatement. To say the least, my parents should have had their parenting license taken away. Before one of my siblings was born, my mother was discovered having an affair with a Sear's salesman, so it's very possible that my sibling is my-half sibling. We've talked about it a few times, and all we do is laugh. It's just another one of our "mother stories." Who cares who fathered whom? Besides, we may be able to get a discount on appliances at Sears. We were always very close and continue to be. I felt that I needed to mother as much as I could as an eleven-year old since my mother was incapable of taking care of this child.

Fortunately, Aunt Winnie, who had raised my mother, was the backbone of the family. Without her God knows where I'd be. Auntie was stable, which was a novelty in my family. She was loving and nurturing, and the only one able to keep my parents in line. For instance, one Thanksgiving Day, our family was planning to have dinner at the Fish and Game Club. That morning, like many other mornings, there was chaos. My mother was in the bathroom, passing "suicide notes" under the door. My father had a handgun in his pocket and threatened to make her wishes come true if she didn't come out and join us for dinner. We then went to the Fish and Game Club, knowing that our father had a gun in his pocket. Needless to say, the turkey dinner didn't go down very well. When we returned home, as was our pattern when things were unraveling at home, my brother and I ran to Auntie's house next door and told her about the gun. Auntie was barely five feet tall and my father was over six feet, but Auntie had the heart of a lion. She immediately marched over to our house, stood toe to toe with my father, and said, "Norman, give me that gun." My father then took the gun from his pocket and handed it over to Auntie who was not to be denied, if you knew what was good for you. Happy frickin' Thanksgiving. That day was pretty much on a par with the day my mother threw the Christmas tree out the front door.

Throughout my childhood, I was sick pretty much all of the time. Mostly it was strep throat. Thank God for penicillin which had just been developed, mainly to treat the wounded in the war. Upon my father's return from the war, he would nightly give me a shot of penicillin. Then the pill came out, and I was spared the nightly jabbing. Even with the penicillin, I still was sick a great deal of the time. What I noticed about my mother was that when I was sick and seeing a doctor on a regular basis, my mother was in her glory. She was the star of the show. The sicker I was, the more dramatic she became. Sometimes I think that she consciously or unconsciously contributed to my poor health so she could have her moments in the spotlight. I was resigned to the fact that I would likely be sickly for most of my life, but when I left home at the age of nineteen, my health gradually began to improve.

In my family there were alliances. There was my mother and my brother, and my father and me. My father taught me how to read when I was four. My father signed my report cards most of the time and chastised me when he thought I could do better. Whenever he went to visit a friend or do an errand, I tagged along. I was grateful for the attention and loved my father for loving me. Then it all fell apart. When I was about ten, my father started to molest me. It started by him slipping into bed with me at night. My mother was there but not there, if you get my drift. This happened in the 1950's when sexual abuse was never talked about. There were no programs in schools that urged sexual abuse victims to tell a trusted person what was happening. There was no sexual abuse reporting law until the 60's. All of us who were being victimized had to suffer in silence which allowed these violations to continue unchecked.

During this time, my father had a small restaurant. He opened the restaurant every morning, my mother then took over, and my father was able to be home right about the time I got home from school. This gave my father a perfect opportunity to raise the bar, which he did. It was the most horrific time of my life. I felt trapped and that was probably because I was. There was no one to tell and nowhere to go. All I could do was pray for it to stop. The sexual abuse was bad enough, but when you love and trust a person who then does the unthinkable to you, the damage is magnified. I lost my father. I lost his love and companionship. I was truly alone and learned well how to be alone. It is something I have had to fight all of my life. I want to be close to people, but I also want to guard myself from the pain of betrayal, and in large measure I have the inability to trust.

I kept this secret until I was thirty-years old and in college when I told a classmate about the molestation. That was the beginning of my efforts to heal and to help others. Years later I worked as a social worker on sexual abuse cases and eventually wrote a book, *How to Claim Your Power*, to help sexual abuse survivors empower themselves and avoid becoming victims in all areas of their lives. I also hoped to break the cycle of abuse, knowing that people oftentimes do to others what was done to them. I had come a long way and was determined to go even further. It had been a long time in coming.

All the time I was growing up, my father drank and drank heavily. Needless to say, our family was always scrambling one way or another. When he was thirty-five, my father had a great deal of his stomach removed due to ulcers. Because his incision became infected, he had to have wires to fasten one side of his stomach to the other. He was in the hospital for a month, and when he was discharged, he began to drink again. My father then was offered a job as a chef in Massachusetts, and we moved there for a time. Because of his drinking, that job didn't last very long. We moved back to New Hampshire and lived with Auntie. Since we were cramped like sardines in a can, my father began to build a house for us to move into. Actually, it was a garage. This was to be a temporary living arrangement as my father had plans to build a house adjoining the garage. However, if you've ever known anyone who would rather drink than work, you'll understand why the house was never completed.

By then I was in high school. I was still precocious but seemed to avoid trouble. Sitting in the principal's office was not something I wanted to repeat. I was a bright kid, but I never applied myself. It took everything I had to survive the instability of my home, or should I say the garage. One thing I excelled in was English. Since my father had taught me to read when I was four, and because the only form of entertainment we had at that time was the radio, I read almost every book in my mother's bookcase.

In my senior year, I had the English teacher who taught all of the college-bound students. I knew I wouldn't be able to go to college since that idea was discouraged by my parents, but I just got lucky by being in that particular English class. Miss Noyes was demanding and expected the best from all of us. We had to write an essay to be turned in every Monday. That was quite a challenge, but Miss Noyes insisted that we complete this assignment. What she did was to get each student to improve their writing skills, and I benefited greatly from this Herculean task. At the end of the school year, all the seniors had the opportunity to enter a writing contest, the winner to receive the Dodge Prize, something that was a feather in the cap of anyone who was lucky or smart enough to win it. Miss Noyes was very competitive, and she was determined that one of her students would win. She made a deal with us. If we would go to the library in lieu of her class once a week, we could work on our papers and be relieved of class. Naturally, we all agreed. It was a no brainer. The girls had to write about wildlife in New Hampshire. We were to pick one insect or animal and write about it complete with footnotes from our research. I chose the honeybee, and I was surprised to find that I really enjoyed leaning all about the life of the honeybee. What I thought was going to be a very boring exercise turned out to be a fascinating study of this creature. The boys had to write about a specific time in the history of New Hampshire. Who came up with these subjects? It sure wasn't an easy assignment.

On graduation night the winners were announced, and I won the Dodge Prize for the female group. I couldn't have been more shocked. After all, I was in a class with kids who were destined to attend schools like Harvard and Wellesley, and I was just a kid who lived in a garage with a crazy family. This award really changed my life. I was never given much encouragement at home or told that I could do something that would cause the family to be proud, and now I competed with the crème de la crème of students and came out on top. It took me quite awhile to absorb my victory, but when I did, I was even more motivated to one day go to college. I was determined to do well, and be recognized for being an excellent student, which I intended to be. However, I first had to find my way out of the garage. College was not an option for me at that time but marriage was.

My first step in my escape plan was to get married at nineteen. At twenty I had my first child, Lori Lynn. I remember the day I was in the hospital holding Lori in my arms and crying tears of, "What do I do now?" Lori's pediatrician came into the room and asked me why I was crying. I told him that I didn't have the slightest idea how to raise a child. He said to me with great confidence and wisdom

"Always follow your instincts, and you can't go wrong." I did just that and managed to do a pretty good job as a mother. Kristen Marie followed three years later, and by that time I was better prepared to raise a child. I had it down pretty good. I was a stay-at-home mom and loved everything about it. However, my marriage was rocky, to say the least.

My husband's job required us to live in Vermont and finally in Massachusetts where I joined a church and became very active. One of the volunteer opportunities I had was to accompany the priest to a local nursing home and assist him when he gave communion to the residents. In those days, a wafer was used to symbolize the body of Christ. Because many of the elderly residents would choke on the dry wafer, someone had to walk behind the priest and give a glass of water to the choking person. It was there that I met Jean. It has been said that you have a friend for a reason, a season, or a lifetime. I've had all three, but I think the lifetime ones are the best. Jean proved to be a lifetime friend, and it all started in a nursing home where I used to refer to me and Jean as "The Communion Rescue Squad." Throughout the years, Jean and her husband, Bobby, have rescued me more than once. Our friendship gave me some respite from a failing marriage, and, along the way, we managed to make some elderly people very happy.

You have not lived until you have
done something for someone who can never
repay you.

-unknown

. . . And the Band Played On

At the time Jean and I were volunteers at the nursing home the band leader, Mitch Miller, was very popular. He had an album called, "Sing Along With Mitch." Jean and I bought various instruments such as kazoos, slide flutes, harmonicas, and maracas, and we would hand them out to "our band." We would start the record player, and Jean would say, "Okay, everybody. Instruments up." Jean and I would march around the room complimenting each person on their musical prowess. I think the residents enjoyed the foolishness of it all. I know Jean and I did. Before we led our band, we would go around to the rooms of residents who were not able to join us downstairs, and visit with them for a few minutes. On time a woman loudly asked us, "Did I eat yet?" I asked the nurse if she had eaten to which the nurse answered, "Yes, she just had lunch." We told the woman, "Yes, you've eaten." Her next question was, "Did I like it?"

Then there was the time when I sat next to a woman to have a chat. She looked as if she had picked off most of her nail polish, but there was still some remaining at the base of her nails. I decided to help her out and finish the job. While I was picking away, a nurse came in the room and said, "Boy, did we have a time with her last night. She had diarrhea, and it was all over her." I guess I wasn't picking nail polish off her nails. Jean has never let me forget that.

The nursing home was an interesting place to volunteer. Elderly people are uninhibited, which I think is one of the best things about getting older. My daughter, Kris, wasn't in school yet, so she came with me to the nursing home each week. Kris was a real tomboy. She always wore jeans and a jersey. Her hair was very long, and she had braids that ran down her back. One day when we were conducting our band, there was a woman in a wheelchair, reciting the rosary. Kris was really into it, and she was shaking her maracas to beat the band (forgive the pun). The woman angrily looked at me and said, "Tell HIM to stop." Then there was Gladys who stole Helen's false teeth. On occasion one of the men would slip into a woman's bed. One day Roy was smoking a cigar and he set his paper bib on fire. A nurse quickly threw a glass of water on Roy to douse the flames. There was never a dull moment.

One of the residents was a guy named Howie. He was mentally challenged and had been in the nursing home for years. He loved to stand outside by the side of the road with a huge grin on his face and wave to everyone who drove by. Jean and I used to call Howie the "Sheriff of Northborough." He loved it, even more so when Jean and I gave him a sheriff's badge. He wore that badge with such pride and really took his job seriously. Of course, his only job was to wave to the passersby, and he did it very well. I don't think he ever made an arrest. He had an unblemished record in that department. Good ole' Howie. He was a great sheriff but a better waver.

Jean and I have memories that go back for many years. We watched all of the Watergate hearings, sitting next to her pool. We planned a fortieth birthday parade for another friend which included forming a marching band. Jean even convinced the high school band leader to lend us uniforms for the occasion. We had a balloon man and a motorcycle that had the lead. We all had instruments which we played very badly, but we proudly marched down the street being led by a majorette. We attracted a lot of attention, sold a few balloons, and really surprised the birthday girl. Jean sure knew how to throw a party.

All the while, my marriage was falling apart, and my husband and I decided to separate. Jean and Bobby were like bookends, making sure I didn't fall over. I was alone during the blizzard of 1978 in New England and was stuck, really stuck in my house surrounded by mounds and mounds of snow. I couldn't have gone to the store for food if my life depended upon it. Being only five feet tall, I probably would have been in snow up to my eyeballs and not be found until the Spring melt. So Jean had her son, David, go to the local market on his snowmobile and get me enough food to sustain me and the two girls.

Jean and Bob were determined to keep me from going into a deep depression. One Christmas time when I was bartending at the Dew Drop Inn, Jean and Bob picked me up after work and the three of us went up the street to the VFW where many of the V's had been celebrating all evening. There was a piano in the hall, so Jean said to the guys at the bar that she was going to play Christmas songs. First Jean played "Silent Night" and then said that she would take requests. Little did the audience know that the only song she could play was "Silent Night." The first request was for "Joy to the World." So Jean proceeded to play "Silent Night." The guys looked confused but assumed that Jean had indeed played "Joy to the World." There were a number of requests, but Jean played "Silent Night" each and every time. Bobby never tires of telling that story. It's his "Silent Night" story.

Then came the divorce. My ex-husband was eager to sell our house as soon as he could, but there were some repairs that had to be made. Bobby immediately went to work and did all the repairs before we put the house on the market. Jean, on the other hand, did everything she could to keep me afloat. I was so overwhelmed. There are friends, *and there are friends.*

The secret to a rich life
Is to have more beginnings than endings.

-Dave Weinbaum

Another Beginning

I had never given up my dream of one day going to college. When both girls were in school, I made my dream come true. I enrolled in Worcester State College, and I don't think I missed four classes in over four years. I was in my element. I loved every minute of it. I used to choose my classes, as much as possible, during the time the girls were in school. When I graduated in 1978 I ranked 29th out of 763 students. I was on my way. After earning my undergraduate degree, I decided to get a master's degree. In one of my classes at school was a husband and wife, Dave and Vida Farrar. We became good friends. One time I shared with them a really awful date I had, but I did it with humor. They loved the story and decided that a single man that they knew would enjoy it too. They asked me if I would be willing to go on a double-blind date. Since I wasn't having much fun at the time, I decided that it would be a good break from school and work. They wouldn't tell me anything about my date, but they said I wouldn't be disappointed.

We arranged a date and time, March 29, 1979, and Dave and Vida along with my date, picked me up at my apartment. Vida asked me how my internship was going at the Westborough Day Hospital, and I told them about some of my experiences. My date, who now had a name, Norm Helm, chimed in and seemed to know quite a bit about psychology which was my major. I asked him if he was a psychologist, and he replied, "Didn't Dave and Vida tell you what I do?" I told him that I didn't know anything about him because

Dave and Vida wanted me to be surprised. He said, "I'm Reverend Norman Helm. I'm Dave and Vida's pastor at the Congregational Church in Westborough." They wanted me to be surprised, and I certainly was. Dave and Vida were determined to be matchmakers, and It didn't take long for us to realize that we were indeed a good match. One Sunday, our friends asked me to go to Norm's church with them. I wore a bright yellow pant suit, and when I was going through the receiving line after church, Norm asked me if I was going to a canary convention; a great combination—a handsome, intelligent man with a good sense of humor. It wasn't long before Norm and I both knew that we loved each other, and began to learn about each other while knowing that our lives were becoming intertwined for good and all.

l learned that Norm had grown up in upstate New York during WW11. Like most families during that time, sacrifices had to be made and times were tough for almost everyone. Money was scarce and housing, if you found it, was marginal. At one time, Norm's Dad bought a building that had once been a barn. There was no insulation, of course, and the winters in New York are brutally cold, so Norm would get up in the morning and see his footprints on the frost on the floor.

Norm was a skinny little German kid who was terrorized by many of his schoolmates because he was German at a time when the United States was at war with Germany. It was a scary and painful time for Norm and something that haunts him to this day. In high school Norm was very bright and a popular student. Even though he wasn't able to read until he was in the third grade, he certainly made up for it. When he finally learned to read, he read voraciously and learned about as much as he could about everything. Norm was curious and loved school, knowing that it was preparing him for the world which he was anxious to join as an adult. After graduating from high school, Norm attended Alfred University, and after he graduated, he decided to enroll in Andover Newton Theological

School. To this day, if anyone asks him why he decided to become a minister, his answer is always, "Darned if I know." After graduating from Andover Newton, Norm's career as a clergyman began.

Norm got married and had two children. The marriage soon began to unravel. Norm's wife had a very demanding job, and Norm was very involved with his work as an assistant pastor and then a senior pastor; not a great formula for a committed relationship. After seventeen years, both Norm and his wife decided to divorce. His ex-wife moved to a city near Boston with the children, and Norm remained in Westborough as senior pastor of one of the larger churches in town.

Norm and I were so grateful to have found one another, however, our time together was interrupted by a sabbatical that Norm was scheduled to take for three months beginning June first. We both agreed that we would resume our relationship once he returned from his sabbatical, but we were dreading the separation. We told each other that we would write or talk on the phone every day, and we did. I think that we became even closer by sharing our feelings in those letters. I kept them all. When I read them it brings me back to a time when our love was new and promised to grow throughout the years. Now people, mainly because of technology, communicate in very different ways. I am grateful that the only way we could stay connected was though our letters and occasional telephone calls. But the letters. The letters.

June 2, 1979

. . . Yes, love. Let's keep our eye fixed on our tomorrows while yet we love today; apart but no less in love.

Gretchen, don't doubt this is real. I love you, and I am not an adolescent. I know what I feel. I know I have never felt it before, and I want to keep feeling it. I have never been more certain about anything in my life. I have wanted to be a grown up, love a grown up and be loved by a grown up, and I have found what I want with you.

I have hardly had time to miss you, but more than that I think I have been protecting myself. It was very painful for me to leave you. It hurt, and it scared me a little. I haven't hurt like that in a long time. In the hallway of your apartment, I thought I would explode! The pain was almost physical, and I was fighting a powerful urge to run back and pound on your door. Now as I remember that some of the pain comes back. I think that is what I have been protecting myself against.

I am trying very hard to simply remember how good it was for those beautiful weeks we had. I don't think I have ever been happier. I just want to keep saying, "I love you" over again. It is, I think, a rare and a beautiful thing to be so childishly in love with maturity. To experience such clean, innocent sweetness of love through my tired, hurt, scared old self is such a blessing; a gift one not often given.

I cannot believe this separation will separate us. I cannot believe we could be so wrong. Surely we both have a firmer grasp on reality then that. I am coming to believe that God is very intimately involved in my life right now, and part of that includes the miraculous fact that we found each other. I'm not at all sure anymore that we found each other so much as we recognized each other when we were brought together.

My love, I am coming to the end of the page and my energy. I love you more deeply than I ever believed possible. Take very good care of yourself. You are my treasure, my pearl.

I love you, Norm

June 3, 1979

Gretchen, I love you. Just now I let the picture of you that I carry in my head come into focus. I have to work at convincing myself that it's not a dream; that you and I really happened. My God, those were fantastic days and nights! They were real, they are real, and there will be more just like them—no better!

I have to tell you everything that I have been thinking and feeling, and I want you to know that my love for you is complete. There are no limitations of commitment or time or duration of anything else. You are everything I have always wanted. I want you in my life, and I want to be in yours—always. I don't ever want to be apart from you like this again.

Please take care of all the good things you are. Live and grow this summer. Be at peace and rest. Take as much into yourself as you can hold and save it all for me, and I will do the same so that when I return we can just pour ourselves into each other. I once told you that I believe that love is something that two people make between themselves out of the feelings they have for each other. When I come home (home is with you), we will make such love, more than we have already known because of all the feelings for each other we have kept these three months.

I love you so much. I wish these days would fly by. I don't want to skip any of them, but I hope they hurry. I want to be back with you. Be at peace and remember, I love you.

Norm

June 4, 1979

. . . I talked with my mother this afternoon. I talked with her about you. I told her how wonderful you are and a little of how in love with you I am.

It is true, Gretchen. I am taking you with me on this sabbatical. It's marvelous. I love you to think of—to write to—to dream of. You are one with me. Gretchen, Gretchen you lovely, warm, funny, delightful woman. I love you. My love, you are so alive, so full of life and no destruction—innocent by choice and wise by experience—a woman a man can love forever and this one will.

I love you. I love you. I love you so. I wrote this. Be kind, English major. I'm in love.

There was a time when all the wounds had closed
Nothing bled, but healing waited;
a slow time when inside things settled at a pace I
could keep,

but living waited.
My bulb rooted itself down
gathered strength
nourished itself deep
but bloom waited, and burst, thrust up into the sun
lived, laughed, loved
finally, fully loved
You.

. . . I love you so much. It is good to be in love; to hear you say, "I love you", to touch you over all the miles; to know you're really there loving me and will be there for me to come home to. You have changed this whole thing for me. You have changed my life. I'm very grateful. I thank God for you are a gift beyond all my deserving. I thank God for us, and I put our love in his care to keep for us.

I love you, love you, love you, and I miss you very much, but my heart is full. Be well my love and at peace.

Norm

June 5, 1979

Gretchen, my love

. . . One of the things I hunger for is a friend that I can talk to about you. I need to tell people about you; this marvelous lady that I have met and fallen in love with. I feel like I have this great secret inside me that I'm just bursting to tell. I want to shout, "Hey, everybody. I'm in love. She's wonderful, kind, decent, bright, pretty, loving, tender, and she loves me!!! Can you believe it? She's all these things and much more, and she loves me, and, of course, I love her. Let me tell you all about it." But I don't. I keep it inside me, and I only take it out at times like these. I need a friend to tell it to.

I stare at your picture and just let my mind slide back to when we were together and forward to when we shall be together again . . . I love you. Over and over again I want to tell you I love you, and my love is growing and deepening even apart from you. Oh, Gretchen don't leave me. Trust me. Trust us. What we have found is real and uncommon and very precious. You are the end of a long and sometimes painful search—someone to be with so completely and intensely yet comfortably. "Home" is the best word to describe it. Wherever you are and I am is home. That is what meeting you has meant to me. Never, ever again will I be apart from you by choice.

There is a hunger that can only be filled by the fruit of one tree;
A thirst that can only be slaked by the water of one well;
A chill that can only be warmed by the heat of one fire.
One tree, one well, one fire, one you.

I love you, darling,
Norm

There are so many more letters and cards, and I cherish them all. Norm returned from his sabbatical at the end of August 1979. We were finally reunited and found that time had only strengthened the bond between us. It was as if we had never been separated. I believe that the three months that we were apart proved without a doubt that we were in love, deeply and without any doubt that we found what we had both been looking for, for a long, long time. It was worth the wait.

Work and play are words used to describe
the same thing under differing conditions.

-Mark Twain

Love, Work and Play

After dating for two years, Norm and I were married September 20, 1981. We decided that given his position as pastor, we could either get married with only our children present or get married in church and invite the entire congregation. We decided on the latter and put invitations in the bulletins one Sunday. One of the members of the church made the wedding cake, and a group of ladies prepared the food for the reception which was to be held in the church hall. It was the beginning for me to get to know people better and for them to get to know me.

Norm was dedicated to his work. He worked as hard as any man could be expected to do, but he never tired of his job. He loved ministering to people, he loved administrative work, and, most of all, and he loved preaching. He married couples, baptized their babies, and conducted many funerals. Thankfully, there were some light moments, and thank God for them. Norm's secretary, Mrs. Ridley, gave Norm something that he put on the wall behind his desk. It said, "Only those who play can truly work." So Norm balanced work with doing things he enjoyed doing. One of those things was fishing with his best friend, Walt. Norm would leave for the pond early in the morning, come home, change into his work clothes which were always a suit, tie, and vest. He was then ready to start the day having had some quiet moments drifting around, and, if he was lucky, catch a few bass which were his favorite fish because those suckers were a real challenge. Norm was a "catch and release" fisherman which means just that; he would catch a fish and release it back into the pond to the great relief of the fish, I'm sure. One time he caught a real whopper. He had a bucket and put the fish into the bucket filled with water. He then drove home when the day was just dawning and woke me up. He said, "Gretch, get the camera. I want to have a picture of this fish as proof that I caught the biggest bass I have ever seen." I took a couple of pictures, he returned to the pond and released the fish, and I went back to bed. A wife has to do what a wife has to do.

Norm was always willing to help whomever needed something, and invariably someone down on their luck would come into his office and ask for money. Norm had a policy of never giving money for obvious reasons (does muscatel ring a bell?). If someone needed a meal, Norm would give them his card and tell them to go to the local diner, give the owner his card and order a meal. Norm would then would go to the diner and pay the owner who had a running tab for such occasions. One time when Norm went to pay for a gentleman's meal, he found that the man had order a lobster salad sandwich and one to go. No flies on that guy.

Another time a man came into the office and approached Mrs. Ridley and asked for money. Mrs. Ridley explained that the policy of the church was not to give money but to assist people in other ways. The man became belligerent, so Mrs. Ridley rang for Norm. Norm immediately responded and asked the man what he wanted. When he said he wanted money, Norm repeated the policy of the church to him. The man persisted, so Norm pointed out the door to him and told him to leave. When leaving, the man turned to Norm, held out a couple of appropriate fingers and said, "Curses on you, you old man." Norm turned to Mrs. Ridley and said, "I didn't mind being cursed, but I sure didn't like being called an old man."

One man that Norm helped each time he needed him had a very horrendous alcoholic life. On one occasion he had fallen asleep too close to a train track. Inevitably the train came, and the poor man lost his arm. After he recovered from his injury, he was given an artificial arm with a hook. From time to time this man felt that he had to enter rehab. The problem was that no one would admit him while he had the hook on his arm. He would always give it to Norm for safekeeping, and when he was discharged, he would get his arm back. Norm used to store this man's arm in the closet in his office. One day, Mrs. Ridley opened the door of the closet to get something for Norm. She saw the hook, looked at Norm and said, "Nothing would surprise me, Mr. Helm."

Over the years there were many times that a person in need was helped. There were many meals provided and even one man needed tires for his car, so Norm sent him to the local tire store, and the man received four new tires. I said to Norm, "What if some of these people are just scam artists looking to get something for nothing?" Norm replied, "That may be true, but if forty-nine people scam me, and I provide something to the fiftieth person who is honest about needing something, then it's all worth it." I was learning an important lesson about the ministry, or at least how one person in the ministry thinks and acts. I guess we all bristle when people try to take us for a sucker, but that didn't bother Norm. He never even gave it a second thought.

Norm had a unique way of looking at religion. He always knew that there were more questions than answers. On one occasion a man, disheveled and in need of a good bath, wandered into the church during the service. He was starting to become somewhat disruptive, so one of the deacons took him gently by the arm and led him out of the sanctuary. After the service, the deacon approached Norm and said, "You know that guy said that he's Jesus Christ." Norm said to him without hestitation, "How do you know he isn't?"

One of the duties of a pastor is to officiate at a funeral. Norm had worked regularly with the local funeral director, Warren Rand, who was a member of the church. One day Warren told Norm that he had to drive to New Jersey with a man who was to be buried in a cemetery with his family and friends present. The one thing that was lacking was a minister. Warren asked Norm if he would be willing to go with him to perform this duty. Norm agreed. The next day, Warren and Norm left for New Jersey in Warren's hearse. Because it was a long distance from Massachusetts, they had to leave very early in the morning. They arrived at the cemetery. Norm greeted the family, expressed his condolences, and conducted the service for the gentleman. When Warren and Norm were heading back home on the turnpike, they came to a toll station. Warren took the ticket and gave it to Norm to hold for him. This had been a long, long day for both of them, so Norm asked Warren if he could stretch out in the back of the hearse and take a nap. All the while he had the toll ticket in his pocket. When Warren drove up to the booth where he was to pay the toll, he told Norm that he needed the ticket. Norm promptly rolled down the window of the hearse and handed the toll collector the ticket. I don't know if that toll collector ever recovered from that incident, but I'm sure he had a strong heart or Warren would have had another customer.

One of the most enjoyable things about being part of Norm's ministry was that every time Norm was asked to officiate a wedding, the couple would invariably tell him that I was welcome to come to the reception with him. He asked the couple to send me an invitation. Norm thought that I should not just be a "tag along" but an invited guest. After word got around that this was the appropriate thing to do, I received an invitation to every wedding that Norm performed. I asked Mrs. Ridley to write in calligraphy the reading from the book of Ruth that Norm always read at the weddings. I then bought some frames, and Norm and I would bring this gift to the reception and place it with the other gifts. The couples were always so grateful to have such a special memento of the wedding, made all the more special because it came from the minister and his wife.

A couple of times I attended the wedding rehearsal the night before the wedding. Norm was adamant about everyone paying attention and not allowing themselves to be distracted. He didn't allow any foolishness, which can occur when people are excited about the upcoming festivities and may have even started celebrating a little early. Norm knew that if everyone paid attention and knew exactly where they were supposed to be and when, the wedding would not turn into a disorganized spectacle. The first time I saw Norm do a rehearsal for a wedding, I was completely taken aback with his intolerance of people who weren't taking things seriously. I told him that I thought he conducted a "Nazi wedding rehearsal." After that all the rehearsals were referred to as "Nazi wedding rehearsals." Norm thought that was pretty funny, and I think he became even more Nazi-ish just to live up to his reputation.

Norm believed that a wedding was one of the most special times in a couple's life, and he made it very clear that there would be no cake smushing on their faces when they cut the cake. In order to reinforce this directive, Norm wrote what he referred to as "the cake ceremony." It said something about the tradition of offering food to a visitor and sharing life with them. He pointed out that the couple would be sharing their lives together and symbolic of that was the sharing of the cake; the sharing of life. Everyone who ever heard "the cake ceremony" was entranced by it. Many people asked Norm if he could give them a copy as a remembrance of such a beautiful part of the reception. The guests seemed to be very grateful that they didn't have to witness such an undignified cutting of the cake and the subsequent cake in the face routine.

Attending every wedding was such a delightful experience. We got to meet many family members whom we had never met before. We always had a wonderful dinner, and we danced, danced, danced. That was quite a surprise to many people. Just hours before Norm was standing at the altar pronouncing a couple husband and wife, and then he was dancing to Glenn Miller and Elvis. One time when we attended the wedding of Walt Temple's niece, Walt's mother, who was not an active church member, saw Norm and me dancing and remarked to Walt, "It kinda' makes you believe in religion, don't it."

One time Norm was performing a wedding ceremony for two very elderly people in the chapel of the church. He asked the gentleman to repeat the wedding vows after him. Norm read the first sentence and waited for the man to respond. Silence. Norm repeated the sentence again. Still silence. Norm was getting increasingly nervous with the situation and at a loss as to what to do next. After he read the sentence for the third time, the gentleman turned to Norm and said, "Oh, I'm sorry, Rev. Helm. I was just being dazzled by the beauty of my bride."

Norm realized early on in our marriage that I was someone who enjoyed have a fun time. I think he realized, too, that doing fun things was just what he needed to take the pressure off his daily grind. He was more than happy to join me in some of my antics. For instance, one Halloween I decided to dress up as a witch (and, no that wasn't type-casting). I put on a black smock, witches hat, and make-up befitting a genuine witch. I also had some organ music playing and a skull candle in the window. I asked Norm to join me in this little escapade, but he refused. After I was all decked out, he decided to change his mind and make this a real scary stop for the trick or treaters. He put on a sweater with a pillow on one side of his back. He put milk of magnesia on his face, and he walked hunched over. Now, he started to orchestrate the plan. He went into the kitchen and put a number of pots and pans and a big spoon on the counter. He then got a cloth bag in which he put a rubber chicken. "So, here's the plan," he said. You open the door, and I'll start to bang the pots and pans in the kitchen. When the kids say, "trick or treat," you say, "I'll have to call Igor." Then I'll walk into the living room and before you hand them the candy dish, I'll pull the rubber chicken out of the bag." Where's Steven Spielberg when you need him.

The younger kids were accompanied by one or both parents, so they knew they were safe from Igor and the witch. At the end of the evening, three teenage boys rang the bell. They stood there in their cockiness, and said, "Trick or treat." That's when the pot banging began, and I told them that I would have to call for Igor. So help me God, they turned as white as ghosts, which was appropriate for Halloween, and one of the boys said in a shaky voice, "Who the hell is Igor?" They finally caught on when Igor pulled the rubber chicken out of his bag. Believe me, they made a hasty retreat. The evening had been a huge success. We saw many cute little costumes and smiling faces, and we scared the crap out of three not so brave teenagers.

One time our daughter, Lori, was living in Phoenix, Arizona and decided to bring her boyfriend home to meet her parents. He asked her if he was expected to wear a suit coat and tie to dinner since he would be dining with the minister and his wife. Oh, contraire, I thought. This offered a great opportunity to have some fun with this young man. I then started to put together the clothes I would wear to the airport when we picked them up. I started with leopard pants. Then I found an absolutely tacky gold top and a headband that matched. Now for the shoes. I got some black sling-back heels. Then for the coup de grace, I had a horrible black rabbit fur jacket to top it all off. Norm was not to be outdone. He went to the Salvation Army and picked up a polyester brown shirt, white tie, and the ugliest jacket ever made. He decided to slick his hair back and wear sunglasses. He was a sight to see.

We had a friend in the parish who was a limousine driver. He not only had a limo, but he had a chauffeur's uniform to match. I told him that we would like to hire him to take us to the airport to pick up Lori and her boyfriend. Bob had a terrific sense of humor and thought it would be a great way to spend an evening. So after taking numerous pictures of all of us in our respective outfits, we headed to the airport. Needless to say, when we walked in, we got quite a bit of attention. No wanting to be impolite, most of the people didn't stare but tried to sneak as many peaks as they could at this rag-tag group. Then our daughter and her boyfriend arrived. The minute Lori saw us, she gasped, "Oh, no. That's my mother and Norm."

Her boyfriend's jaw hung open, and I thought that if he didn't close his mouth real fast, it might freeze that way.

Unfortunately, some months later Bob became very ill. Towards the end, Norm planned to visit Bob after the Sunday service. I was very fond of Bob, so I asked his wife, Ginny, if I could go with Norm. She said that of course I could, and that Bob would be very happy to see me. After Norm had talked to Bob and prayed with him, I stood by his bed and talked to him. I asked him if his daughter would be coming to see him. He said that she would be flying in that afternoon. I asked him if he wanted me to pick her up at the airport. Remembering our last airport fiasco, Bob laughed, which was wonderful to see, and he said, "Absolutely not."

Although the pastor is always number one in the church, I was very happy to be the pastor's wife. As a youngster, I attended church regularly. The church was a safe place for me, and I found it to be the refuge I needed. At that time, I was a member of the Methodist Church. Later, having married a Catholic, I converted so that I could go to church with my family and not remain on the sidelines. After my divorce, I also divorced the Catholic Church. I floated around for a while, but when I married Norm, I felt like I was back home. Loving the church as I did, I had the opportunity to be very supportive of Norm which I believe was very helpful to him as he had a very demanding job. Being the pastor's wife gave me a great deal of latitude in getting many projects off the ground. For instance, after I became a social worker I saw that the only toys we offered to our "kids" at Christmas time were second-hand toys. These toys were donated by people who would never give toys in this condition to their own children, so I started an "Adopt a Child for Christmas" program. People would take a child's name from a Christmas tree in the church hall and would buy this child something from the child's wish list. The hall eventually was filled with wrapped presents which we delivered to the office of social services and the social workers delivered them to their "kids" by Christmas. This program was a huge success and continued for many years and may still be going strong.

One of the things I did that I was most proud of was starting a fund to create an accessible bathroom. The church had already installed an elevator, a new sound system, and had large print hymnals available. I thought that we could then put up a sign that signified that we were an accessible building. Norm informed me that it wouldn't be possible to do that because one thing we lacked was an accessible bathroom. I saw this as a necessary project, but it was one that was not greeted very well by the trustees. They believed that the amount of money it would take to make an accessible bathroom a reality would cost up to $100,000. I wasn't deterred. We held a "Goods and Service Auction" where we made $3,500 which was a good start. I was also a member of the Congo Mama's Dirt Band. This started as a one-time event for the Women's Fellowship but was so well received that we were asked by other churches to entertain for them. We charged a nominal fee, and all the proceeds went towards the bathroom fund.

Norm was now eligible for another sabbatical. He had dreamed of spending those three months in Israel but thought that since we had a mortgage to pay, it was "the impossible dream." Many people in town knew of Norm's desire to spend his sabbatical in Israel, so one day a realtor approached us and said that she knew of a couple from New Zealand who were coming to the states for their son's wedding. They needed a place to stay for three months, and would we be willing to rent our house to them. The impossible had been made possible.

Norm and I spent three months of his sabbatical at The Tantur Institute for Ecumenical Studies. It was located between Bethlehem and Jerusalem. Bus service went to both towns, so we were able to spend time on the Jerusalem and the Bethlehem buses. This way we were able to learn more about the people and their culture. When we took the bus to Jerusalem, the men were generally dressed in suits and ties, and the women wore dresses or blouses and skirts which was very traditional garb for them. Not so when we took the bus to Bethlehem. Many of the women wore ankle-length dresses, and the men were usually in their work clothes. The bus driver always had some Arabic music playing, and people would oftentimes bring chickens or other animals on the bus. One time a man brought on a goat. Nobody blinked an eye; nobody but me and Norm. There was constant chatter and laughter. Frankly, I preferred the Bethlehem bus because you never knew what would be on board, and it was always a very lively and fun experience.

While at Tantur, Norm was working on a very complex Bible study program and would spend most of the day in the library, typing away. I, on the other hand, had been struggling with my dissertation and still didn't have a date for my hearing. I told Norm that since his writing came so easy to him, he should enroll at Andover Newton Theological Seminary and earn his doctorate. Upon our return to the states, he did just that.

So now we were back to our normal lives, having returned to Massachusetts. A truly fortunate thing happened while we were in Israel. Our friend, Walter Temple, knew of my desire to have an accessible bathroom in our church. Walter was a carpenter by trade, and he managed to find the architectural plans for the building and searched for ways to make that happen. He found that the kindergarten room had two bathrooms. Walt said that he didn't think that young children needed two bathrooms when we could co-opt one, and he was able to convince the trustees of that fact. So Walter went about knocking out a wall and doing all that was necessary to outfit the bathroom to fit the standards of an accessible bathroom. It just so happened that this project cost exactly what we had raised so far—$10,000. Upon our return to the states we returned to our beautiful and essential bathroom for the handicapped.

So life was good and filled with all good things. Our family was happy and healthy. It was 1989, and we were all looking forward to

Christmas. The ladies of the church were preparing for the yearly Christmas Fair which the townspeople always looked forward to. The children were rehearsing for the Christmas pageant. It was a joyous time of the year. And then . . .

Expected the Unexpected

-Roger Von Oech

. . . It Happened

December 1, 1989. Norm was walking home after being in his office preparing to conduct a funeral. It was a lovely, crisp December day. Crossing the street in a crosswalk, he was hit by a car. He was transported by helicopter to UMASS Medical Trauma Unit. He had suffered a massive head injury. The doctors treating Norm had doubts that he would survive such a horrific injury. They did all the things they needed to do to save his life, and they managed to save him against all odds. From the hospital he went to a rehabilitation hospital for three months and then home. It was as if our lives were written on a blackboard and someone took an eraser and erased it all. We now needed to pick up the chalk and to start writing our new lives.

Norm tried to return to being the pastor of the church but was unable to perform all the duties that were a necessary part of the job. We then left Westborough for New Mexico. We lived in New Mexico for fifteen relatively normal years, but for a few years before we decided to move to North Carolina, Norm started to show signs that his traumatic brain injury was taking its toll. He couldn't complete jobs he started. He wasn't able to drive without putting both of our lives in danger, and his short-term memory was becoming increasingly worse. All the while I was in complete denial that Norm was anything but Norm at his best. I covered for him many times. I didn't want to believe that Norm was drifting away.

While our children pointed out the changes in Norm's behavior, I made excuses and refused to accept their observances as real.

We moved to North Carolina to be closer to our children, and Norm continued his decline. The drastic change, I believe, pushed Norm over from traumatic brain injury to dementia. His behavior became unpredictable, dangerous, and he required much more care than I was able to give him. I became depressed and suffered tremendous anxiety. My hands shook so that I could barely sign my name. When I wrote to someone, I had to use the computer because my writing would be illegible. Eventually my doctor prescribed anti-depressants and anti-anxiety medication, but I was in a deep, deep hole. I found a therapist who helped me deal with all the upheaval in our lives, but I continued to believe that life as we had known it had come to an end. I didn't even consider moving on. I felt that everything was over. I was over.

The newsman, Dan Rather, said, "If all the difficulties were known at the outset of a long journey, most of us would never start out at all." I began to dwell on the past, particularly the magical days when Norm and I started to date and then marry. I felt as if I was closing the door on everything. I didn't recognize it at the time, but in retrospect I believe that I was becoming suicidal. I didn't have a plan to end my life, but my behaviors certainly were leading me in that direction. I started to eat less and less. My stomach was churning all the time, so food was not something I wanted even though I probably needed nourishment more than ever. Eventually, I lost all of my appetite and even looking at food or smelling it repulsed me. When we had company for dinner, I would just move the food around on my plate and hope that nobody noticed that I had as much on my plate at the end of dinner as when we started. Sometimes someone would notice and tell me that they didn't think I was eating enough. I assured them I was.

I felt very much as anorexics feel about food, however, my feelings were not about choice but about trying to fade away. After a while

I realized that I had to eat if I was to survive. A small part of me was fighting to go on with life even though I wanted all the pain to end once and for all. I began to buy cottage cheese, knowing that I needed protein even in small amounts. I would choke down a few spoons of cottage cheese each day, but my appetite was still non-existent. I just ate to live.

This continued for too long. When we finally moved to Maryland after almost three years in North Carolina, a friend, knowing that I was having difficulty eating, suggested that I get a protein drink and at least have that during the day. In Maryland, I had all the support I didn't have in North Carolina. I had family and friends who relieved me of the burden of caring for Norm who was only getting worse, but by then I had joined Norm in his illness. I was as sick in my own way as he was in his. I couldn't accept the fact that our lives would never be the same, that we would never return to Westborough, never be part of the church where we had so much life going on. People urged me to move on; to take care of myself, but I couldn't envision a future, especially one without Norm. Because of the dementia, Norm was there but not there. Every time I looked at him, I felt that I was looking at a man who was gone and would never return. In a sense, that was the reality of the situation.

Dementia is a cruel illness. The German word Seele means both psyche and soul. In ancient times, some believed that the soul resided in the brain. When the mind is taken from you, your soul resides somewhere else, inaccessible and unavailable. I felt that I had lost part of myself when I "lost" Norm. I grieved every day for that loss. I needed to move on, but I remained immersed in my pain and confusion. What had happened to us? What was going to happen to us? The fear and doubt I had left me immobilized. I continued to decline along with Norm. You've heard the expression: "The blind leading the blind." Well, with me it was "The sick taking care of the sick." All the pep talks in the world that I got on a regular basis from our children did little to cause the situation to change.

Then everything did change. Norm entered assisted living right about the time we were both on the edge where even the slightest thing would push us over. I experienced many feelings. The first thing I felt was relief. All my time had been devoted to Norm. Towards the end of Norm's living at home, I had a service called "Visiting Angels" which allowed me to leave Norm in someone's care for four hours a week; hardly enough time to do much of anything. However, those four hours were a godsend.

I was finally relieved of the job of caring for Norm. Now he would have "the village" care for him, and I could return to being his wife and not his caretaker, but it left a tremendous void in my life. Everything came to a screeching halt. I worried about the care he was being given. Was he treated well? Was the staff sensitive to his specific needs? Was he upset about not being in his own home with me to be with him each and every hour? I would experience such tremendous anxiety when I would visit him, however, it didn't take long for me to see that he was being taken care of by caring, knowledgeable people who, when they got to know Norm, enjoyed him tremendously. He had retained his sense of humor and his quirky way of looking at things, and he brightened everyone's day. When a member of the staff would ask how he was, he would always reply, "It depends who you ask." After a while, when Norm would ask the staff members how they were, they would respond, "It all depends who you ask."

All of the stimulation, stability, security of assisted living enabled Norm to improve. He had a routine each day that never deviated. He got up at the same time, was assisted in bathing and dressing, ate breakfast and lunch at the same time every day. Seven days a week I would visit Norm after lunch. We would go to the activity room and sit together on a couch. He would read, and I would do word puzzles or read. Sometimes, when the weather permitted, we would take walks in the garden and sit, shaded from the sun by umbrellas. It was such a beautiful place to spend a few hours each day.

Norm was in the perfect place for him, but I was alone; alone with my two very old dogs. The loneliness I felt was awful. After visiting Norm, I would cry all the way home. I knew that we had worked very hard to get Norm into an assisted living facility, and I was grateful that we had succeeded, but our relationship was reduced to visitations of two hours a day. I felt as if I had lost half of myself. I felt as if my life as I knew it had come to an abrupt halt. I missed Norm tremendously, but I wouldn't want to return to caretaking him at home for anything. It was a mixed blessing. He was where he needed to be. I knew that in my head, but my heart was broken, having lost my companion of so many years. I tried to keep a positive attitude. When I was feeling low, I started to count my blessings to that I wouldn't continue a downward spiral. It was a challenging task.

After some time had passed, and I had adjusted as Norm had to the schedule, spending time at the assisted living facility was an enjoyable part of my day. Seeing Norm improve, breathing a sigh of relief that he didn't decline as we believed he would, and brought a lot of comfort to me. Our visits were always delightful. When I would leave, I would hug Norm, give him a kiss, and tell him I loved him. He would respond in the tenderest way, "I love you too, Babe." For the first time in years, I felt as if we were living a normal life. It wasn't what we had planned. It wasn't a normal life in the sense that we were living together and doing all the things that married couples do, but it was a new normal. It was much more than I expected, and I was very grateful to be given more time with Norm; time that was spent enjoying each other's company. The black cloud over our heads had finally given way to lovely rays of sunshine.

Too often we underestimate the power of touch,
A smile, a kind word, a listening ear, an honest
Compliment, or the smallest act of caring, all of which
have the potential to turn a life around.

-Dr. Felice Leonardo Buscaglia

Love Blooms in an Unexpected Place

At first, seeing Norm in assisted living and then returning home alone, was excruciatingly painful. I oftentimes asked myself why I was subjecting myself to such terrible feelings when I could be enjoying the peace and serenity I had lacked for so long. The answer was always that I knew Norm loved the fact that he saw me on a daily basis and that it was contributing to his improvement. Having someone familiar to interact with, especially someone you love and who loves you is such a tremendous part of the healing process.

Spending many hours a week at the assisted living facility, I got to see firsthand how the residents were cared for. I thought about how apprehensive I had been when Norm was first admitted. Since I had done volunteer work in a nursing home many years ago, I had seen firsthand how impatient and even harmful some of the staff members were to the residents. Gradually, I came to see what wonderful care all the people were getting at this facility. No one ever raised their voice or chastised a resident, and this was not an easy population to work with. Everyone on this particular floor had some form of dementia, and some of them were experiencing end-stage dementia, which is the most difficult form to deal with. However, I saw caring, professional people doing the best job they could to make everyone feel special and never neglecting anyone's needs. It was a heartwarming thing to see, and gave me such increased faith in humanity because of these people. The world can be a cold place, but in this place there was warmth and even joy where you would least likely expect it.

I had the opportunity to observe the daily life of this assisted living facility. I was in the middle of all that went on. I came to know the staff personally and considered them my friends. There were people from an outside agency also that were responsible for working with some of the residents who needed physical and speech therapy. Norm badly needed both when he returned from a brief stay in the hospital followed by rehabilitation hospital. I watched them painstakingly and with great patience work to get people walking and communicating. I became particularly fond of a young man who was a physical therapist. Ira was the kind of person who lit up not only the room but the building when he was present. He had a million dollar smile and a heart to match. I always loved sharing a few minutes with him when he came to work with residents. We talked about some of the humorous things that went on. Having worked with abused and neglected children and their families for five years as a social worker, I knew how necessary it was to enjoy the light moments in order to keep going and maintain one's sanity. Burnout is prevalent among people who work with a needy population. We never laughed *at* the residents but laughed at some of the things they said and did.

At this facility, there were times during the day when the staff tried to engage the residents in things such as trivia games, crafts, word games and anything else that would provide stimulation and help the residents to keep their minds active. One day, one of the staff members put up a white board. She told the residents that she was going to put up dashes that represented something with which they would be familiar. She put four dashes on the board. She then said, "It's an animal. It lives in the woods, and it likes to eat fish." Silence. Again: It's an animal, it lives in the woods, and it likes to eat fish." Silence . . . until Ms. Robertson shouted out, **"Would you please give us a clue?"** Again, she repeated, "It's an animal. It lives it in the woods, and it likes to eat fish." One of the residents, to the relief of the staff member, shouted out: "It's a bear." Finally, the answer.

One of the things I saw was that some of the residents had some faithful visitors: sons, daughters, husbands, children and extended family, but many of the residents never had visitors. The only human contact they had was with the staff, who, knowing all too well that families avoided their loved ones for reasons of their own, tried to bridge the gap. I knew that they did their best to make sure that these residents had some form of human contact, but they also knew that they were only substitutes.

I talked to one of the staff about this issue, and she shared with me that sometimes a family member would visit and would say that they just couldn't bear to see their loved one in the condition they were in. The person they once knew was no longer there. The love that was once reciprocated was lost in the vast wasteland of dementia. It was easier to stay away and to rationalize that once the family member was gone, everyone in their former life was gone too. Sadly, this robbed the dementia patient of the loving touch of another human being. They rarely heard the voice that they had heard for many years before dementia set them apart from their loved one.

There were times when I visited Norm when one man, obviously missing human interaction, would walk behind us and vicariously soak up whatever we shared. I knew he was lonely, and I felt compassion for the fact that he didn't have the partner that Norm had. I knew that he was not a threat even when he followed us into Norm's room, but it felt creepy. I used to think of him as a stalker. The strange thing about it was that before I started to do Norm's laundry at home, Norm's clothes got mixed up with his, and he would walk behind us, wearing Norm's shirt. Finally, I got the shirt back, but I wasn't able to get over this man joining us in tandem. Sadly, sometimes when I was leaving and saying goodbye to Norm with a hug and a kiss, he would stand nearby and probably imagine what it would be like for him to have the affection that we shared.

It was very sad to see so many people forgotten by their families. I came to know some of them during my visits, and I always tried to acknowledge them and to ask how they were. It was not much, but it was at least something in addition to the attention they got from the staff. The more I saw this, the more I was convinced that I was doing the right thing by visiting Norm every day. More and more, I was able to drive home after leaving Norm without crying. I understood, all too well, why family members resisted visiting their loved ones in assisted living, but I still felt that it was important for them to rise above their painful feelings for the sake of the person who was living alone with dementia.

Norm was fitting in very well. When I would walk into his room, he would say, "You're home." I would answer, "Yes, I'm home." I was so relieved that Norm considered his assisted living facility his home because, in actuality, it was. Walking down the corridor, he would stop and talk to one of the other residents. He never lost his willingness to reach out to people. There were times when he carried on some very normal conversations with me. During those times, I would tell myself that he really didn't belong in assisted living, especially in a dementia unit. Then he would say something like, "I was worried about you being in Argentina last night." I would remind myself once again that Norm was doing as well as he was because he was in assisted living. On occasion when I would take him out for a brief trip to the library or to our daughter's house for dinner, he would become disoriented. Change was confusing to Norm. Change scrambled everything in his brain, and he wanted to return to where he felt that everything was normal. Once he returned to assisted living, he was less anxious and felt that he was where he belonged.

All the tension and fatigue that I had experienced for the past few years was beginning to dissipate. I was able to get a good night's sleep. I wasn't worried about Norm because I knew that he was being well cared-for. I still felt a void in my life, living alone, having a very limited social life, but I was beginning to adjust. Past experience taught me that you can get used to anything if you endure it long enough and develop a positive attitude. Norm and I seemed to be growing ever closer. Both of us were able to be with each other each day, and we cherished the moments we spent just relaxing and enjoying each other's company.

I was slowly getting on with my life. I still had my two old dogs to keep me company, but that was to change, as I knew it would in the not too distant future. Skout was about fifteen or sixteen-years old. Having gotten him from the pound when he was about a year old, we could only estimate his age. Our daughter, Kris, brought Pooh Bear to us when he wandered into her UPS building one rainy night, and she brought him home, having no other option. He was about fourteen-years old and having difficulty with his right legs. I tried everything I knew to do to give his legs the support they needed, but all my efforts were in vain. I took him to an orthopedic vet who recommended testing to determine if he had a genetic condition, but it turned out that he was just suffering the ravages of old age.

One morning I found Skout in the kitchen unable to get up. At the end of the day, when nothing had changed, I called our vet and was told to bring him in, and they would see what they could do for him. Kris and I put Skout in a clothesbasket, wrapped in a blanket, and we went to the vet; both of us anticipating the worst. The vet had looked at Skout's records and saw that he had an enlarged heart. She asked us what we wanted to do, and we knew what we had to do for Skout's sake. We said our goodbyes, through tears and hugs, and left without our much loved companion. We contacted a cremation service, and a week later, I picked up Skout's ashes in a lovely box with an engraved plate that said: Skout Helm—To know him was to love him and everyone did.

Thirteen days later, I had to make the same decision for Pooh Bear. By this time, he could barely stand up, and I knew that his time had come. Pooh Bear, unlike Skout, hated to go to the vet's. He would start whimpering as soon as he got through the door, and it was a real challenge to treat him because he resisted with all of his seventy pounds. Kris found a mobile veterinary unit, and one afternoon a lovely, caring young woman came to the house. She remarked that Pooh Bear certainly was a magnificent looking dog, but she also stated that she knew we were making the right decision. My neighbor, Eileen, who is an animal lover extraordinaire, joined me and Kris. Pooh Bear's passing was done with him on his own bed, surrounded by his loving family and the neighbor who had cared for him when I traveled to Connecticut one weekend. Although I was heartbroken to lose him, it was such a relief to see him finally at peace. His ashes are alongside those of Skout's and our first dog, Caillech.

So now I was alone. My lease at the house I was renting was to expire in about a month, so now I had many more options since I didn't have any pets. I found a lovely apartment and began to weed out so many things that we had carried around with us for years. This was truly going to be a new start for me. I would be closer to Norm and our daughter and her partner. I bought new furniture. I didn't want to transport the past with me. I kept only those things that were of sentimental or utilitarian value. Everyone told me that I needed to move on with my life. It was not what I had planned or what I expected, but, then again, sometimes in life unexpected things happen.

Being loved by someone gives you strength,
while loving someone deeply gives you courage.

-Lao Tzu

The Promise

I'm a life-long liberal and proud of it. I'm a women's rights, civil rights, Social Security, Medicare, Medicaid, Head Start, food stamps, pro-union, clear air, clean water, safe food, safe workplace, "Ask not what your country can do for you," end of legalized racial segregation and gender discrimination, liberal. If you're gay, that's okay. If you're gay and want to get married, you have my blessing. Just tell me where you want me to send the wedding gift. I'm pro-choice, but I would never have an abortion. That's my choice. I believe that children need to be able to grow and to choose their own paths in life as unfettered as possible, but in my house there were strict rules of behavior (curfews, zero tolerance of drugs, emphasis on learning which always requires oversight of the parents, to name a few.) These are my values although some like to believe that liberals are without values. I happen to believe that liberals are all about family values. But that argument is for another day. Let me just repeat that I'm a liberal and proud of it.

How can I be a liberal and believe that living together without the benefit of marriage is not something that I would support? Don't get me wrong. I don't think living together vs. marriage is a moral issue. I'm not in the least qualified to pass judgment on the morality of others. No, my objection is both pragmatic and realistic. When two people make the decision to live together, they have no rights as a couple under the law. If the coupling comes to an unhappy end, there's no basis on which to decide who gets what, including, most importantly, the children and pets. Everything depends upon the reasonableness and fairness of both parties. Sometimes it works out well. Other times it's a nightmare. It's all up to the two people involved who, hopefully, are not angry, vindictive or bitter. Although legally bound couples still go through the agony of divorce which involves lawyers and the court that is responsible for dissolving the contract, it is still my belief that a legal marriage is still preferable to one that is not.

This is why I come down strongly on the side of marriage vs. cohabitation because I believe that marriage whether it is between heterorsexual or homosexual couples is the best way to go through life with your life partner. I will be accused of being old-fashioned and betraying my liberal ideology, but, for me, marriage brings with it a promise, a promise that is tremendously important and meaningful. It defines the relationship in a committed and important way when a couple makes a promise or a vow that they, hopefully, will honor for the length of days they have together. It is the base on which everything rests and something that each person in the relationship can hold onto when their marriage is tested, sometimes in brutal and trying situations. The vows, which are often said in the context of a religious ceremony and in a church, don't have to be seen as religious and don't need to be said in a church, although most times a church is the setting for the marriage of one person to another. The vows themselves are not religious in nature although many people view them as such and that's their prerogative. They are simple, straight-to-the-point statements that carry tremendous weight and define more than any other words spoken, what marriage should be.

These are the words I spoke and the promise I made when I married Norman Helm in 1981:

> I, Gretchen, take you, Norman, to be my husband, to have and to hold from this day forward, for better or for worse, for richer, for poorer, in sickness and in health,

to love and to cherish; from this day forward until death do us part.

Forty-six words; only forty-six, but they constitute a promise that brings with it great meaning and oftentimes requires great strength to honor. They are not to be taken lightly. There are times when I never think about the promise I made. Then there are times when I repeat those words over and over again to myself to reinforce that I made a promise and intend to live up to that promise no matter what circumstances make it difficult My word is my character, and to keep my word defines who and what I am and what I stand for. When Norm was hit by a car and suffered a traumatic brain injury, the neurosurgeon said that he had the worst head injury he had ever seen in anyone who survived. Needless to say, the process of healing required tremendous stamina and determination. Norm has often said that while his injury demanded a lot from him, it didn't come close to what this family and friends had to endure. The accident left Norm with short-term memory loss, loss of concentration and focus. In addition to all the losses we had to endure, one of the most painful one was Norm's inability to be the pastor of his church and to be part of the ministry that be loved so much and did so well. I also had to give up my plans to be a family counselor. I had just earned my doctorate in psychology after working for many years to earn it, but Norm needed my help and there was never a question that his needs superseded mine.

. . . for better or for worse.

Then after seventeen years of living with this disability it morphed into dementia. Dementia is unpredictable and takes away a person's ability to live a normal life. Being the caretaker of someone with dementia is a demanding, never-ending job. Each day you are faced with watching your loved one fade away into a place that is not accessible to you. Norm suffers from confusion, delusions, loss of the memory of people and places, and any other facet of human behavior that he used to depend upon to navigate the world. Norm was not able to drive. He had to depend upon me to bring him wherever he needed to be. He couldn't be left alone for any period of time so that meant that my life had to be lived in tandem with his until he entered assisted living.

. . . in sickness and in health.

The vows that we made many years ago have special meaning now because we are living them. Of course, there are couples who never took those vows who are as faithful and caring to their partners as I am to Norm, but for me, my fidelity to the words that I spoke with such conviction give me strength. Who knows why? I just know that when they were spoken, they were written on my heart.

A promise made. A promise kept . . . until death do us part.

Love is a friendship set to music.

-E. Joseph Cossman

Dear Gretchen,

Nobody has ever been more a part of me and my life than you have been and are; nor have I ever known anybody as well and as deeply as I know you. We are not one; we are a pair—one helluva pair!

Because you are you and I am me, we don't march in lockstep—we dance; freely, improvising as we spin around this floor of life. I much prefer dancing for the dance itself than marching to get someplace.

So, just hold me, and we'll dance at least another nineteen years.

I love you,
Norm

Written by Norm to me on the occasion of our nineteenth wedding anniversary.

One of the nicest things you can say to your partner,
"If I had it to do over again, I'd choose you. Again."

-unknown

I do . . . Again

I have never wanted to renew my marriage vows. There are some people who like to mark a special occasion such as a wedding anniversary with a renewal ceremony, but it was never something that appealed to me. Then Norm and I were about to celebrate our thirty-year wedding anniversary. Our relationship had undergone some significant changes such as Norm being in assisted living while I lived alone, visiting Norm for only two hours a day. It wasn't exactly the ideal marriage, but, in some ways, it was. Norm had improved greatly since being in assisted living. He had a regular routine. He was safe and secure. The staff made every attempt to engage him and to make sure that he was well cared for. For all these reasons, and many more, Norm was a lot better than before he entered assisted living.

We were very close and our relationship was stronger than it had ever been. I talked to our friend, Rev. Martin, and told her that I thought that a renewal of our vows ceremony was something that I had considered. I told her that I certainly wouldn't want to proceed if Norm was not in agreement or able to understand what we were doing. I hoped that we could plan the ceremony and scrap the plans if Norm was not well enough to participate. Rev. Martin agreed that it was a good idea. When Norm and I married nearly thirty-years ago, our vows were a promise for the future. After thirty years, having been challenged numerous times, our marriage had become a promise fulfilled.

I talked to Norm about renewing our wedding vows, and he thought it was a good idea and would love to commemorate our thirty-year wedding anniversary that way. From time to time, I would ask him questions such as, "Would you like to marry me again?" to that question he responded, "I'll think about it." I said, "Well, you'd better make a decision before I order the cake." With that, he kissed my cheek and said, "That's my answer." Our anniversary would be September twentieth, but our daughter, Lori, and our grandchildren, Parker and Brooke, were coming to Maryland to visit so we decided to have the ceremony while they were here. I asked Parker if he would do a reading, which he agreed to do, and I asked Brooke to be my maid of honor. We set the date for Saturday, July twenty-third at 1:30.

I asked the assisted living facility if we could have the ceremony there. They were delighted and said that they would do anything that they needed to do to make it happen. I told them that all we needed was the use of the activity room. I told them that I would extend invitations to the residents on Norm's floor and also the staff. I ordered flowers and a cake. I made invitations that I gave to everyone. Many of the staff members were excited about the idea and planned to attend. The day was fast approaching.

One of the residents, Ms. O, as she was called, wanted to help on the day of the ceremony. I was happy to have her help me and to also help her feel needed. So many of the residents had lived very active lives before entering assisted living, and I think they missed the many things they were used to doing. Even though their minds and bodies were not one hundred percent, they longed for the lives they once had when they felt important and necessary. Growing old has its advantages, but it also has its downside.

July twenty-third I picked up the cake and the flowers. It felt very much the way it did thirty years ago when Norm and I were married. I was nervous but very excited about having such a wonderful day to share with our friends, family, and Norm's fellow-residents. Rev.

Martin stayed with us in Norm's room until it was time for the ceremony to begin. At 1:30, she walked out of the room with us walking behind her, arm in arm. I had picked a lovely song by Barbra Streisand, "If I Never Met You" which was playing while we walked down the hallway, which to me felt like walking down the aisle. The residents and our family were seated in the room. Parker and Brooke stood at each corner. Before the ceremony was to begin, Rev. Martin said that she had something to say. First, she welcomed everyone and thanked them for coming to share this lovely occasion with us. Then she said:

Over the years I have officiated at numerous weddings. I have performed weddings for the young and the older. I have no idea how many of those marriages begun still exist. Perhaps I would be surprised if I knew which ones made it through all the complications of life.

The ones that I would have predicted would fail would be the ones who overtly ridiculed the wedding vows and obviously were not taking them seriously. Over the years I have come to understand that almost anyone taking those vows really do not understand the depth of their meaning until they begin and continue to live their lives together. Even with pre-marital counseling, the depth of the meaning of the words "love", "comfort", "honor", remain with in "sickness" and in "health", "be faithful" are elusive until actually experienced. All too often life is random and unexpected as well. Sometimes marriages just can't stand the challenge.

Looking forward to a healthy, happy life together, Norman and Gretchen first took these vows nearly thirty years ago. A happy normal life was rudely and violently interrupted when Norm was the victim of a reckless driver. He barely survived. His brain was damaged. The accident affected not only Norm but Gretchen, the whole family and their friends. Norm couldn't continue with his ministry. Gretchen gave up her career. All were affected.

But life did not stop. Through sickness and health, there remained comforting and loving and honoring. Sometimes it seemed that hell was bursting out all over. Sometimes there was a rainbow at the end of the storm. Life went on. The years went on and changed them both positively and negatively. Sometimes the silence was deafening. But, through it all, because of inward strength and God's guidance, because of the pure determination and purposefulness of all who have supported and loved this couple, the birds, once silent, would be heard singing again. Here we are today to celebrate. We celebrate and renew vows once taken, and so honored and kept that they are an example for us all. The human spirit powered by God's generous grace gives us the sure knowledge that in the end love, held close and true, does triumph.

A gift of love for Gretchen and Norm,

Rev. Dr. Donna J. Martin

We were so moved by Rev. Martin's words and her affirmation that we had honored and kept our wedding vows even under the most trying of circumstances. Then Parker was asked to do his reading. First, he said some very lovely things about both me and Norm. This was unexpected but appreciated immensely. Parker read a short piece written by Ruth Reiche:

Marriage is a vow to encourage each other to realize their own best qualities. You believe that you have found a person who will stretch our own limits, one who will provide a constantly challenging dialogue to encourage each person to grow in their own direction.

You do not come to marriage to find a resting place.

Then it was my turn to say something. After all that had been said thus far, I hoped I could maintain my composure. Having read what I had written to Norm on our twentieth anniversary numerous times, I always shed a few tears, however, I knew that I had to try to be unemotional, as hard as that would be. I said:

Norm,

Going through some papers, I found something that I had written to you on the occasion of our twenty year wedding anniversary ten years ago. I want to read it to you now, and to let you know that I meant what I said twenty years ago, and mean it more today as we celebrate thirty years together.

I read:

Happy Anniversary
September 20, 1991

> Norm,
>
> It has been twenty years today and somehow I can't believe it. It has gone by so quickly. It reminds you that you should savor each day because someday you will look back and wonder where all the time went.
>
> Our time together has been filled with a lot of life. We've had many obstacles to overcome many challenges to face together, and many glorious moments. The important thing is that we've done it all together. Somehow that has made the tough times easier and the good times more sweet. If I had to choose a partner, which I luckily did twenty two years ago, I couldn't have chosen anyone better.
>
> You are loving and supportive. You listen to me and counsel me. You are there when I need you and not there

when I don't. You tread so easily through my life and even in the worst of times, I never felt that you or our relationship was a burden. It has not always been easy, but it has always been worth it.

My hope is that we are given many more years to be together to love each other, to love the life we've made. With you by my side, I greet each day with joy and wish that everyone could know the love and friendship we have. We have learned that in the midst of the uncertainties of life and in spite of our flaws and imperfections, we can live a life that is exciting yet peaceful, stable but dynamic, alone yet very much a part of the world.

I love you, Norm, more now than when we began our life together. I can't imagine living a day without you in my life. I hope this milestone is just the first of many and that our years together will continue to be as happy as these first twenty have been.

Love,
Gretchen

We then repeated the wedding vows we had said to each other when our life together began. After the ceremony, we cut the cake, sharing it with each other and with everyone else who was in attendance. It was a wonderful gathering of family, friends, and Norm's fellow residents in assisted living. There was a lot of life going on that day. There was a lot of gratitude that this day had come to pass. Some months earlier when Norm was in the hospital and very sick, his doctor said that he would never be able to return to assisted living but would have to be in a skilled nursing facility for the rest of his days. At that time, I talked to Rev. Martin about conducting a memorial service for Norm when he passed, which at the time seemed imminent. This day, the day of our renewal service, it was

Rev. Martin who presided over the service. Was it an irony or a miracle—probably a little of both.

So we continue to love one another, to share our lives together, being grateful for each day . . . and dancing.

But I'm still having an interesting life.

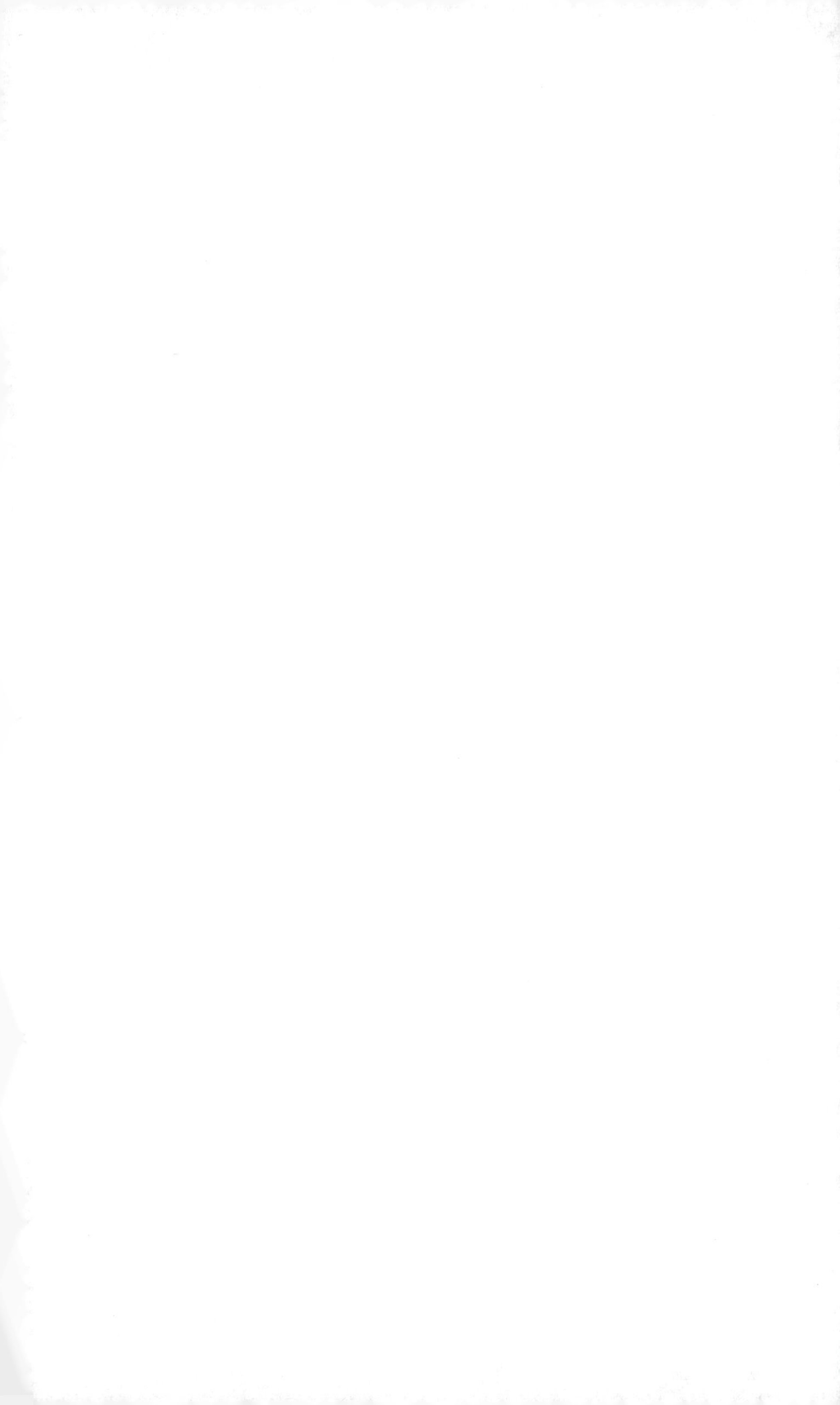

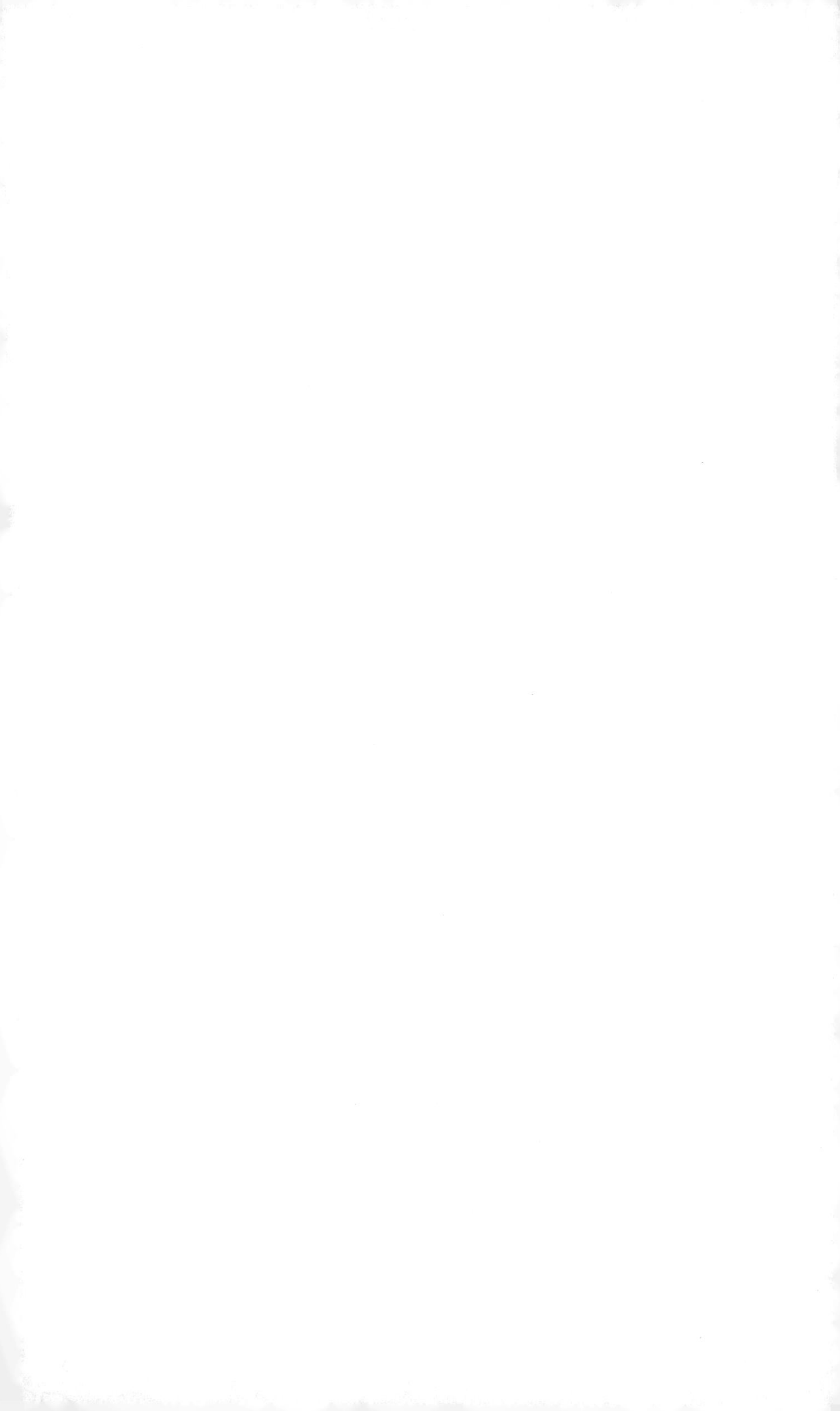